NCLEX: Perioperative Nursing

103 Practice Questions & Rationales to EASILY Crush the NCLEX!

Chase Hassen

Nurse Superhero

© 2015

Disclaimer:

Although the author and publisher have made every effort to ensure that the information in this book was correct at press time, the author and publisher do not assume and hereby disclaim any liability to any party for any loss, damage, or disruption caused by errors or omissions, whether such errors or omissions result from negligence, accident, or any other cause.

This book is not intended as a substitute for the medical advice of physicians. The reader should regularly consult a physician in matters relating to his/her health and particularly with respect to any symptoms that may require diagnosis or medical attention.

All rights reserved. No part of this publication may be reproduced, distributed, or transmitted in any form or by any means, including photocopying, recording, or other electronic or mechanical methods, without the prior written permission of the publisher, except in the case of brief quotations embodied in critical reviews and certain other noncommercial uses permitted by copyright law.

NCLEX®, NCLEX®-RN, and NCLEX®-PN are registered trademarks of the National Council of State Boards of Nursing, Inc. They hold no affiliation with this product.

© Copyright 2015 by Chase Hassen and Nurse Superhero. All rights reserved.

Have you seen my other NCLEX Prep Books?

NCLEX: Respiratory System : 105 Nursing Practice Questions and Rationales to Easily Crush the NCLEX!

NCLEX: Endocrine System : 105 Nursing Practice Questions and Rationales to EASILY Crush the NCLEX!

NCLEX: Cardiovascular System : 105 Nursing Practice and Rationales to Easily Crush the NCLEX!

NCLEX: Emergency Nursing : 105 Practice Questions and Rationales to Easily Crush the NCLEX!

EKG Interpretation: 24 Hours or Less to Easily Pass the ECG Portion of the NCLEX!

Lab Values: 137 Values You Know to Easily Pass The NCLEX!

First, I want to give you this FREE gift...

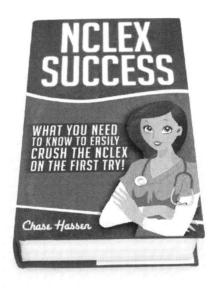

Just to say thanks for downloading my book, I wanted to give you another resource to help you absolutely crush the NCLEX Exam.

For a limited time you can download this book for FREE.

http://bit.ly/1VNGAZ9

Table of Contents

First, I want to give you this FREE gift... _____ 4
Chapter 1 : NCLEX: Perioperative Questions _____ 6
Chapter 2 : NCLEX: Perioperative Questions, Answers, and Rationales _____ 58
Conclusion _____ 110
Highly Recommended Books for Success _____ 111

Perioperative Nursing

Chapter 1 : NCLEX: Perioperative Questions

The following are 105 questions that will help you study for the NCLEX evaluation. All of the questions are based on things you might need to know in the area of Perioperative Nursing. Following the quiz will be the identical questions with the answers and rationales. Compare your answers with the correct ones to see where you may need to study some more. Good luck!

PLEASE NOTE: The answers are located in the next chapter. If you would prefer to see the questions and answers as you review this study guide, visit page 58.

1. A preoperative assessment on a client is being done. What is included in the perioperative assessment? Select all that apply.
   a. Dietary preferences
   b. Previous hospitalizations and surgeries
   c. Allergies
   d. Signed surgical consent
   e. Pain score
   f. Electrolytes

Answer:

2. The most important nursing intervention in a preoperative client is what?
   a. The client's level of pain
   b. The preoperative EKG
   c. The identification band is in place
   d. The client's blood type is noted

Answer:

3. Which client is at an increased risk for surgical complications?
   a. A 24-year old with mild asthma
   b. A 90 year old male with heart disease
   c. An 18-year old female who is overweight
   d. A 34 year-old female with fibromyalgia

Answer:

4. Diabetics are at special risk for surgical intervention because of what reason?
   a. They need a light snack before surgery to manage their blood sugars.
   b. They have an increased risk for deep vein thrombosis.
   c. They need modification of their medication regimen on the day of the procedure.
   d. They have a higher risk of respiratory complications.

Answer:

5. A client is extremely anxious prior to their procedure. What do you say to the client?
   a. Being anxious is common. You will feel better when the procedure is over.
   b. Extra medication can be given to you to allay some of your anxiousness.
   c. Most people don't die of surgery so you have nothing to be worried about.
   d. Try to relax. The procedure is only in a moment's time.

Answer:

6. What medication should be reported to the surgeon if the patient has been taking it up to the point of surgery?
   a. Ibuprofen
   b. Digoxin
   c. Dyazide
   d. Tylenol

Answer:

7. What is the most worrisome sign for a nurse to note in a preoperative evaluation?
   a. A history of peripheral edema.
   b. A history of allergies to betadine.
   c. Recent chest pain on exertion.
   d. A history of mild asthma.

Answer:

8. What should the preoperative nurse teach the client about the postoperative phase? Select all that apply.
    a. The postoperative diet
    b. Deep breathing and coughing exercises
    c. Postoperative exercise of the lower extremities.
    d. The removal of dentures.
    e. Pain control techniques.
    f. The skin preparation.

Answer:

9. What is included in the preoperative checklist?
    a. Dietary restrictions.
    b. Verification of signed surgical permit
    c. Preoperative pain medication
    d. The teaching of splinting the incision

Answer:

10. Complications of the intraoperative period include what?
    a. Hypoxia
    b. Elevated body temperature
    c. DVT
    d. Hypercoagulability state

Answer:

11. The client is to have regional anesthesia. What do you tell the client about this type of anesthesia?
    a. The client will be intubated.
    b. A local anesthetic will be injected along the pathway of a nerve.
    c. The client will have no memory of the surgery.
    d. The surgery will take longer than with general anesthesia.

Answer:

Perioperative Nursing

12. The client is undergoing conscious sedation. How do you explain this to the client?
    a. There will be a better ability to tolerate unpleasant procedures while conscious.
    b. Intubation is performed after the sedation is given.
    c. No local or regional anesthesia is necessary.
    d. The client does not need an anesthetist present for the procedure.

Answer:

13. The client is having local anesthetic for their surgery. How do you explain this to the client?
    a. The area along a nerve route will be anesthetized.
    b. The client will have a shorter procedure with local anesthesia.
    c. The client will have no memory of the procedure.
    d. The anesthesia will involve the area around the surgical site.

Answer:

14. The nurse tells the client about the main complications of anesthesia. What does she say? Select all that apply.
    a. Bronchospasm
    b. Hypertension
    c. Dysrhythmias
    d. Fever
    e. DVT
    f. Prolonged pain

Answer:

15. What is the best way to reduce infection during surgery?
    a. Use povidone iodine topical solution to the affected area
    b. Give antibiotics after surgery
    c. Keep the wound free of dressings
    d. Provide adequate oxygenation

Answer:

16. The client is undergoing conscious sedation. What things should be monitored? Check all that apply.
    a. The peripheral circulation
    b. Vital signs
    c. O2 saturation
    d. EEG
    e. The placement of the ET tube
    f. Level of consciousness

Answer:

17. You are the operating scrub nurse. What is a major part of your job?
    a. Assess level of consciousness
    b. Assess vital signs
    c. Perform instrument, sponge, and needle count
    d. Assess body temperature of client

Answer:

Perioperative Nursing

18. You are the circulating nurse in a surgery. What are some tasks you might do? Select all that apply?
    a. Manage the airway
    b. Do a sponge count
    c. Open sterile supplies
    d. Contact the post-anesthesia recovery room
    e. Assist in retraction
    f. Provide assistance for the scrub nurse

Answer:

19. You are the postoperative nurse assigned to patient care after surgery. What is your priority nursing intervention?
    a. Contacting the relatives about the surgery.
    b. Maintain a patent airway.
    c. Check the surgical dressing.
    d. Assess peripheral pulses.

Answer:

20. The client is suffering from postoperative laryngospasm. What is a priority nursing intervention?
    a. Turn the client on his side.
    b. Check the vital signs
    c. Intubate the client
    d. Suction the airway of irritating secretions

Answer:

21. A medication given to treat postoperative laryngospasm includes what?
    a. Inhaled racemic epinephrine
    b. Albuterol
    c. Fentanyl
    d. Corticosteroids

Answer:

22. As a postoperative nurse, you note that the blood pressure is 20 percent less than the baseline preoperative blood pressure. What is suspected?
   a. Effects of pain on the postoperative client
   b. The giving of Fentanyl during surgery
   c. Hypovolemia from surgical blood loss
   d. Hypothermia during surgery

Answer:

23. You note a significant decrease in the client's postoperative blood pressure. What is a good first nursing intervention?
   a. Check the incision site
   b. Give extra fluids for resuscitation
   c. Turn the client on his left side
   d. Place the client in a semi-Fowler's position

Answer:

24. A common cause of postoperative hypertension in a client is what?
    a. Pain
    b. Increased O2 sat
    c. Dysrhythmias
    d. Anesthesia complication

Answer:

25. The client has sinus tachycardia after surgery. What do you suspect is wrong?
    a. The patient has had an MI.
    b. The patient is suffering from a normal complication of anesthesia.
    c. The client is in pain.
    d. The client is being given too much O2.

Answer:

26. The client has sinus tachycardia after surgery. What do you do as the postoperative nurse?
    a. Reduce the IV rate.
    b. Treat the underlying cause.
    c. Give epinephrine.
    d. Place the client in a Trendelenburg position.

Answer:

27. The client is suffering from sinus bradycardia after surgery. What is the most likely cause?
    a. Effects of general anesthesia.
    b. High spinal anesthesia
    c. Hyperthermia
    d. Acute MI

Answer:

28. The client is suffering from sinus bradycardia after surgery. What is the medication of choice?
    a. Bretylium
    b. Epinephrine
    c. Atropine
    d. Norepinephrine

Answer:

29. The client is suffering from hypothermia after surgery. What is a nursing intervention?
    a. Check the vital signs
    b. Apply warm blankets
    c. Increase the IV fluids
    d. Increase client activity

Answer:

Perioperative Nursing

30. The client is suffering from postoperative agitation. What is the first thing the nurse must rule out?
    a. Hypoxia
    b. Hypothermia
    c. Arrhythmia
    d. Anxiety

Answer:

31. The client is suffering from postoperative nausea. What should the nurse give the client?
    a. Increased fluids
    b. Zofran
    c. Atropine
    d. Increased O2

Answer:

32. The client is at risk for gastric aspiration after surgery. What is the main risk factor for this condition?
    a. Conscious sedation
    b. Surgical pain
    c. Hypothermia
    d. Tracheal intubation

Answer:

33. A common pain control method used in the post anesthesia recovery center is the following:
    a. Massage
    b. Meditation
    c. Patient-controlled anesthesia
    d. Succinylcholine

Answer:

34. The postoperative client is suffering from hypovolemia. What signs or symptoms might be present? Select all that apply.
    a. Bradycardia
    b. Tachycardia
    c. Hypertension
    d. Hypotension
    e. Cardiac arrhythmia
    f. Cool skin temperature

Answer:

35. The postoperative client has suffered from an evisceration. What is the first nursing intervention you should consider?
    a. Replace abdominal contents
    b. Apply a sterile moist dressing to cover the affected area
    c. Increase IV fluids
    d. Turn the client to the left side

Answer:

36. Which postoperative finding is least worrisome?
    a. Urinary output of 30 cc/hr
    b. Respiratory rate of 20
    c. Blood pressure of 80/40
    d. Pulse of 120

Answer:

37. The postoperative client has absent bowel sounds. What should the postoperative nurse do?
    a. Feed a solid meal slowly
    b. Feed liquids only
    c. Ask for permission to put an NG tube down
    d. Give a retention enema

Answer:

38. The postoperative COPD client has an O2 Sat of 87 percent. What do you do?
    a. Talk to the anesthetist about reintubating the client.
    b. Give 100 percent O2 by rebreather mask
    c. Give albuterol
    d. Give 2-4 liters of oxygen by nasal cannula

Answer:

39. The client after surgery is at risk of deep vein thrombosis. What can you do?
    a. Ambulate the client in the post-anesthesia unit
    b. Give IV heparin
    c. Apply compression stockings
    d. Ask about inserting an intravenacaval filter

Answer:

40. The nurse recognizes that which of the following drugs might place the surgical client at risk for perioperative complications?
   a. Acetaminophen
   b. Aspirin
   c. Omeprazole
   d. Diphenhydramine
   e. Ibuprofen
   f. Zoloft

Answer:

41. Which of the following items should be included when teaching a client about an upcoming outpatient procedure?
   a. Postoperative nursing interventions
   b. Risk for postoperative complications
   c. Risks and benefits of the proposed procedure
   d. Risks and benefits of anesthetic choices

Answer:

42. You are reviewing the chart of a client about to undergo general anesthesia. Which of the following is the greatest risk factor?
    a. The client who expresses anxiety about the procedure.
    b. The client who ate a snack within the last three hours
    c. The client who last smoked 24 hours ago
    d. The client who has hypertension controlled by diet and exercise

Answer:

43. What is a priority nursing assessment when caring for a preoperative client?
    a. Ask about allergies.
    b. Verify client identity.
    c. Determine the client's nutritional status.
    d. Determine the client's neurological status.

Answer:

44. The nurse is obtaining a history from a client at risk for malignant hyperthermia. Which of the following should the nurse assess first to get the most accurate risk assessment?
    a. Previous history of surgical complications.
    b. Drug allergies.
    c. OTC drug use.
    d. History of unexplained fevers.

Answer:

45. The nurse is worried about a client's risk for impaired gas exchange because of ineffective airway clearance. What is a priority assessment?
    a. Respirations per minute
    b. Liters of oxygen used
    c. Decreased air movement
    d. Capillary refill

Answer:

46. The nurse cares for a postoperative client after general anesthesia. Which is a priority observation that should be reported immediately?
   a. Complaints of nausea
   b. Mild hypertension
   c. Decreased urinary output.
   d. Increasing body temperature.

Answer:

47. You are caring for a client who is perioperative. What is a priority nursing intervention to prevent infection during surgery?
   a. Preparation of the skin site.
   b. Maintaining hemodynamic status.
   c. Maintaining client temperature
   d. Determining estimated blood loss

Answer:

48. The nurse is caring for a client receiving conscious sedation. What is the priority item to be regularly monitored?
    a. Temperature
    b. Level of consciousness
    c. Dermatome level
    d. Urine output

Answer:

49. What should the perioperative nurse monitor in evaluating ineffective thermoregulation?
    a. Cardiac rhythm
    b. Blood pressure
    c. O2 saturation
    d. Temperature

Answer:

50. Which is a priority nursing intervention in a postoperative client?
    a. Establishing a patent airway
    b. Maintaining adequate blood pressure
    c. Following level of consciousness
    d. Assessing pain level

Answer:

51. The client is postoperative. Which would indicate that the client has a compromised airway?
    a. A complaint of anxiety
    b. A complaint of pain
    c. A pulse oximetry reading of 90 percent
    d. Cool and clammy skin

Answer:

Perioperative Nursing

52. The postoperative client has a compromised airway. What is a priority nursing intervention for this?
    a. Reposition the client to be supine.
    b. Open the airway with a chin lift or jaw thrust.
    c. Prepare to intubate the client.
    d. Notify the surgeon.

Answer:

53. What nursing measures are important in the prevention of laryngospasm?
    a. Administer atropine
    b. Reposition the client to be supine
    c. Administer high flow oxygen via mask
    d. Administer succinylcholine

Answer:

54. The client is immediately postoperative. What would alert the nurse that the client is becoming hypovolemic?
   a. Diastolic blood pressure of 100 mm Hg.
   b. A complaint of severe pain.
   c. A complaint of anxiety.
   d. A blood loss of 500 cc.

Answer:

55. The postoperative client develops sinus tachycardia. What is a good nursing intervention?
   a. Give warm blankets.
   b. Give atropine.
   c. Position the client in a lateral position.
   d. Manage the client's anxiety.

Answer:

56. The client has become hypothermic after surgery. The first nursing action would be what?
    a. Position the client in a lateral position.
    b. Give an analgesic.
    c. Remove wet clothing.
    d. Monitor intake and output.

Answer:

57. The client is confused just after coming out of anesthesia. What is essential in determining the cause of the confusion?
    a. Check the airway.
    b. Check the cardiac rhythm
    c. Check the level of consciousness
    d. Assess the level of anxiety

Answer:

58. The nurse is seeing a client prior to surgery. What is a specific risk factor for aspiration?
    a. Obesity
    b. Cigarette smoking
    c. An elevated sodium level
    d. A history of sleep apnea

Answer:

59. Which of the following is a priority for a client who has abdominal surgery and complains of pain after surgery?
    a. Monitor the blood pressure
    b. Teach the client how to splint the abdomen
    c. Reposition the client to be more comfortable
    d. Ask the client to describe the pain

Answer:

60. A teenage client has a history of anorexia nervosa. The nurse preparing the client for abdominal surgery is most concerned about the clients risk for what?
    a. Aspiration
    b. Infection
    c. Hypovolemia
    d. Tissue perfusion

Answer:

61. A client is scheduled for a surgery related to cancer exploration. The client has tears in his eyes. What would be a good nursing intervention?
    a. Contact the surgeon to alleviate the client's concerns
    b. Ask the client to describe his feelings
    c. Medicate with an analgesic
    d. Tell the client there is nothing to worry about.

Answer:

62. The client is having emergency surgery for bowel obstruction. What is the client most at risk for in the perioperative period?
   a. Infection
   b. Electrolyte imbalance
   c. Aspiration
   d. Airway obstruction

Answer:

63. The client in the post anesthesia care unit after abdominal surgery complains of feeling a pop and a gush of warm fluid coming from the incision site. The nurse concludes it is from a wound dehiscence. Priority nursing interventions include what? Select all that apply.
   a. Place the client in the supine position.
   b. Get a set of vital signs
   c. Cover the wound with a sterile dressing
   d. Apply O2 at 8 l/min
   e. Contact the surgeon
   f. Increase the IV fluids

Answer:

Perioperative Nursing

64. A client has a patient-controlled analgesia machine ordered. The best time to start the PCA pump is when?
    a. When the client complains of pain
    b. When the client arrives after surgery
    c. Just prior to transfer to the floor
    d. When the client shows evidence of nonverbal signs of pain

Answer:

65. Which of the following tasks can be assigned to the licensed practical nurse?
    a. Informing the client scheduled for surgery about the procedure.
    b. Instruct the client scheduled for surgery on the preop preparation.
    c. Get an informed consent from the client.
    d. Administer a preoperative intramuscular medication.

Answer:

66. The postoperative client is ready to be discharged to the floor. What is a sign that the client has an adequate cardiac output?
    a. Cold, clammy skin
    b. Pale mucus membranes
    c. Normal blood pressure
    d. Pulse of 40

Answer:

67. The postoperative client has tenderness in the calf and swelling of the calf. What is the most appropriate nursing intervention?
    a. Apply compression stockings.
    b. Give subcutaneous heparin.
    c. Inform the surgeon.
    d. Watch for further findings.

Answer:

Perioperative Nursing

68. The postoperative client is complaining of nausea. What does the nurse do?
    a. Notify the surgeon
    b. Give Zofran as ordered.
    c. Increase O2 to 8 liters per minute
    d. Turn the client to the side.

Answer:

69. The postoperative client is complaining of incisional pain. What is the first nursing intervention?
    a. Assess the level of pain on the pain scale.
    b. Give IV morphine.
    c. Contact the surgeon.
    d. Change the incisional dressing.

Answer:

70. What is the most important thing to have in place before entering surgery?
    a. Signed permit for surgery
    b. Client's dietary preferences
    c. History of past surgeries
    d. IV

Answer:

71. What does the client say to indicate that he is ready for discharge from the postoperative recovery area after having general anesthesia to home?
    a. "I will drive very carefully toward home".
    b. "I can return to work later this day."
    c. "I do not need to follow up with my surgeon."
    d. "I have the surgeon's number in case I have complications."

Answer:

Perioperative Nursing

72. What is appropriate to teach the client about pain relief after discharge from surgery?
    a. Continue the opioid pain reliever until the bottle is gone.
    b. Use non-pharmacological measures of pain control as the incision heals.
    c. Take NSAIDs for pain as soon as the client gets home.
    d. Take more opioid medication if the pain suddenly worsens.

Answer:

73. What is a priority for the postoperative patient do in order to prevent pneumonia?
    a. Drink fluids only to prevent aspiration.
    b. Ambulate shortly after surgery.
    c. Use an incentive spirometer after surgery.
    d. Lie in a semi-Fowler's position.

Answer:

Perioperative Nursing

74. Each of the following tasks can be given to an LPN as part of intraoperative care. Select all that apply.
    a. Teaching incentive spirometry to the client.
    b. Monitor vital signs
    c. Obtain informed consent.
    d. Teach wound care to the client.
    e. Monitor intake and output.
    f. Assist with turning, coughing, and deep breathing.

Answer:

75. The patient is being discharged to home. What indicates the client has understood the oral and written instructions?
    a. "I will take more antibiotics if the wound is reddened or is draining."
    b. "I will take my temperature if I feel warm."
    c. I will inspect the wound twice daily."
    d. "I will not lift anything heavy for 48 hours after going home."

Answer:

76. The client needs nutritional advice before leaving the hospital after surgery. What advice do you give?
    a. Limit protein to less than 1 g/kg/day of body weight.
    b. A calorie restricted diet can be resumed if it was ongoing before surgery.
    c. Increase zinc to 4-6 mg/day
    d. Drink up to 1000 cc of fluids per day.

Answer:

77. The alcoholic client is being discharged from same day surgery. What do you advise the client to do around drinking behaviors?
    a. Taking medications with alcohol is acceptable.
    b. Go back to drinking what they had been drinking prior to surgery.
    c. Do not drink after surgery.
    d. Report signs of alcohol withdrawal syndrome to the physician promptly.

Answer:

78. You are discharging an elderly client after surgery. What should you warn the client most about?
   a. There will be an increase in wound infections.
   b. There will be decreased ability of the kidneys to get rid of opioids.
   c. There will be a decreased risk of fever.
   d. There will be an increased perception of pain.

Answer:

79. The client is Muslim and faces surgery to remove body parts. What do you do to discuss this with the client?
   a. Tell the client it is hospital policy to discard body parts that are removed from the body.
   b. Reassure the client that diseased body parts will be left in the body.
   c. Listen to the client's concern about removal of body parts.
   d. Get a written consent for surgery that includes removal of body parts that are diseased.

Answer:

80. What is part of the informed consent for surgery?
    a. Consequences of failing to follow surgeon's orders.
    b. Risks and benefits of surgery.
    c. The name of the anesthesiologist involved in the surgery.
    d. The signature of the surgeon.

Answer:

81. What is important about getting the informed consent for surgery?
    a. The informed consent can be gotten after the client has had a sedative.
    b. The informed consent can be gotten after surgery if the client has had sedation.
    c. The LPN can get the informed consent prior to surgery.
    d. The informed consent must be gotten before the client has had sedation.

Answer:

Perioperative Nursing

82. For what is informed consent not required?
    a. For the giving of oxygen during surgery.
    b. For the disposal of body parts during surgery.
    c. For the donation of organs after death.
    d. For photographing the client during surgery.

Answer:

83. A minor is having heart surgery. What is true of giving informed consent?
    a. The minor may give consent if he or she is above the age of 16.
    b. The minor may not give any informed consent.
    c. The minor may give informed consent if he or she demonstrates understanding of the consent papers.
    d. The minor may give informed consent if he or she has not been sedated.

Answer:

84. Which of the following measures are nursing responsibilities when a client is having surgery?
    a. Develop an individualized plan of care.
    b. Serve as the client's advocate.
    c. Call "time out" if a potential error is observed.
    d. Communicate the outcome of the surgery to the family.
    e. Collaborate with the healthcare team.
    f. Order the client's sedative.

Answer:

85. The client is to have elective surgery. The nurse should plan with the client to schedule the surgery:
    a. If the client wishes to have the procedure done
    b. At the client's earliest convenience.
    c. Within the next two weeks.
    d. Within the next 2 days.

Answer:

86. The client is to be NPO for at least 8 hours before having same day surgery. You learn that a client had a half glass of juice 3 hours prior to admission. What should you do?
   a. Report the incident to the nursing supervisor.
   b. Inform the surgery department.
   c. Notify the anesthesiologist.
   d. Reschedule the surgery.

Answer:

87. The client is anxious before surgery. As the preoperative nurse, you should do what?
   a. Give an anti-anxiety agent.
   b. Describe the procedure to the client.
   c. Reassure the client about the surgeon's capabilities.
   d. Encourage verbalization of feelings.

Answer:

88. The client is receiving atropine prior to surgery. What is the intended outcome of this medication?
    a. Constrict the pupils.
    b. Stimulate the central nervous system.
    c. Decrease cardiac output.
    d. Suppress oral secretions.

Answer:

89. The client is receiving Tagamet prior to surgery. What is the intended outcome of giving this drug?
    a. To decrease volume of gastric secretions.
    b. To decrease the pH of gastric secretions.
    c. To reduce the amount of anesthetic needed.
    d. To dispel unpleasant sensations around the procedure.

Answer:

90. The client arrives in the operating room wearing two post earrings on each eyebrow. What should be done?
    a. Ask the client to remove the earrings and place them in a labelled container.
    b. Call a nurse on the med-surge unit to remove the earrings and give them to a family member.
    c. Remind the anesthetist to remove the earrings when the client is anesthetized.
    d. Secure the earrings with paper tape.

Answer:

91. The nurse notices that a cart brought to transport the client has a nonfunctioning clasp on the safety belt. What should be done?
    a. Call the Safety/Security Department to report the problem.
    b. Use a draw sheet to secure the client during transport.
    c. Contact the engineering department to repair the clasp.
    d. Request a new cart with a functioning clasp.

Answer:

Perioperative Nursing

92. The surgeon is checking the x-ray of a client who is in the operating room for a lung lobectomy. The nurse notices that the name on the x-ray is not that of the client's. What should the nurse do?
    a. Call the x-ray tech to take another x-ray.
    b. Call the surgeon aside to ask to have the x-ray checked.
    c. Look for the correct x-ray.
    d. Call a time out.

Answer:

93. The client is receiving a large volume of packed RBCs during surgery. The nurse should observe the client for hypocalcemia because:
    a. Extra calcium is needed during stressful events.
    b. Anesthesia causes hypocalcemia.
    c. Hypo-perfusion to the parathyroid glands affects calcium levels.
    d. The preservative in packed red blood cells binds with calcium.

Answer:

Perioperative Nursing

94. The client had a partial gastrectomy 24 hours ago and has a nasogastric tube in place. The expected outcome of using a nasogastric tube after a partial gastrectomy is what?
   a. To assess the pH of gastric secretions.
   b. To remove stomach contents.
   c. To delay peristalsis until healing takes place.
   d. To assess the characteristics of drainage at the anastomotic site.

Answer:

95. Three days after a cholecystectomy, a client states that he feels like his stomach is going to burst. He is taking a regular diet. After determining the vitals are stable, in which order does the client do the following to help the client?
   a. Position the client on the right side.
   b. Offer 120 cc of hot liquids.
   c. Auscultate the bowel sounds.
   d. Encourage ambulation.

Answer:

Perioperative Nursing

96. The nurse sees that the client is restless during the immediate postoperative period. What should the nurse do first?
    a. Give a sedative.
    b. Offer ice chips.
    c. Give oxygen.
    d. Apply wrist restraints.

Answer:

97. A nurse listens to the client's breath sounds on the fourth postoperative day and hears a loud, low-pitched, rumbling sound on expiration. What should the nurse do first?
    a. Give oxygen.
    b. Encourage coughing.
    c. Request an order for incentive spirometry.
    d. Reposition the client to a high Fowler position.

Answer:

98. During the extended postoperative period after an abdominal hysterectomy, the nurse notes a urine output of 20 cc/hr. What should the nurse do?
   a. Consider this to be normal.
   b. Evaluate the client's fluid intake.
   c. Prepare the client to be returned to the operating room.
   d. Consult the urologist.

Answer:

99. On the first day after abdominal surgery, the nurse notices an absence of bowel sounds. What should the nurse do first?
   a. Encourage the client to use the patient-controlled analgesia pump more often.
   b. Ask another nurse to validate the findings.
   c. Encourage the client to take more ice chips.
   d. Document the findings in the client's medical record.

Answer:

100. Before nonemergency surgery, the client needs to give informed consent. Which of the following is the responsibility of the nurse?
   a. Obtain informed consent.
   b. Explain the surgical procedure.
   c. Verify that the client understands the consent form.
   d. Inform the client about surgical risks.

Answer:

101. The nurse is verifying that the client has given consent for surgery. For the consent to be valid, there must be adequate disclosure of which of the following? Select all that apply.
   a. Nursing care plan in the post-anesthesia care unit.
   b. Purpose of the proposed treatment.
   c. Risks and benefits of the surgical procedure.
   d. Outcome of the surgery.
   e. Side effects of anesthetics.
   f. Name of the anesthetist.

Answer:

Perioperative Nursing

102. The nurse receives a call that a client is being transferred from the post-anesthesia recovery unit to the floor. What should the nurse do first when the client arrives?
a. Assess the patency of the airway.
b. Assess the drains in the client for patency.
c. Check the dressing for bleeding.
d. Compare the vital signs with those in the post-anesthesia recovery unit.

Answer:

103. A client has undergone lab work prior to getting surgery. Which lab value should the nurse report to the surgeon as it might result in delay of the procedure?
a. Sodium of 141 mEq/L
b. Hemoglobin 8 g/dL
c. Platelets 210,000 mm3
d. Creatinine 0.8 mg/dL

Answer:

Great Job! On the next chapter, you will see the questions you just answered plus the answers and rationales! I hope you did well!

Chapter 2 : NCLEX: Perioperative Questions, Answers, and Rationales

The following are the same questions you just took with the answers and rationales. Compare your answers with the correct answers to see where you may need to study further.

1. A preoperative assessment on a client is being done. What is included in the perioperative assessment? Select all that apply.
   a. Dietary preferences
   b. Previous hospitalizations and surgeries
   c. Allergies
   d. Signed surgical consent
   e. Pain score
   f. Electrolytes

Answer: b. c. d. In a perioperative assessment, previous hospitalizations, previous surgeries, allergies and a signed surgical consent form should be included. The nurse does not need to know the clients dietary preferences nor is a pain scale yet necessary. Electrolytes may be on the chart but are not a part of the nurse's perioperative assessment.

2. The most important nursing intervention in a preoperative client is what?
   a. The client's level of pain
   b. The preoperative EKG
   c. The identification band is in place
   d. The client's blood type is noted

Answer: c. The most important nursing intervention in a preoperative client is that the identification band be in place. The other things are of lesser importance in the preoperative period.

3. Which client is at an increased risk for surgical complications?
   a. A 24-year old with mild asthma
   b. A 90 year old male with heart disease
   c. An 18-year old female who is overweight
   d. A 34 year-old female with fibromyalgia

Answer: b. Clients at extremes of age are at a higher risk with general surgery. The others have a minor risk of surgical complications.

4. Diabetics are at special risk for surgical intervention because of what reason?
   a. They need a light snack before surgery to manage their blood sugars.
   b. They have an increased risk for deep vein thrombosis.
   c. They need modification of their medication regimen on the day of the procedure.
   d. They have a higher risk of respiratory complications.

Answer: c. Diabetics should remain NPO but should have a modification of their medication regimen on the day of their procedure. They are not at an increased risk of DVT or respiratory complications.

5. A client is extremely anxious prior to their procedure. What do you say to the client?
   a. Being anxious is common. You will feel better when the procedure is over.
   b. Extra medication can be given to you to allay some of your anxiousness.
   c. Most people don't die of surgery so you have nothing to be worried about.
   d. Try to relax. The procedure is only in a moment's time.
   e.

Answer: b. You can help the client with extra support but assuring them that extra medication is available will help them recognize you know the seriousness of their feelings.

6. What medication should be reported to the surgeon if the patient has been taking it up to the point of surgery?
   a. Ibuprofen
   b. Digoxin
   c. Dyazide
   d. Tylenol

Answer: a. Ibuprofen is an NSAID that can affect the blood coagulation at the time of surgery. It must be withheld for the week prior to surgery. The other medications can be taken up until the time of surgery.

7. What is the most worrisome sign for a nurse to note in a preoperative evaluation?
   a. A history of peripheral edema.
   b. A history of allergies to betadine.
   c. Recent chest pain on exertion.
   d. A history of mild asthma.

Answer: c. A history of chest pain on exertion could indicate significant cardiovascular disease which would put a client at risk for surgery. The other signs are less concerning and another antiseptic can be used instead of betadine.

8. What should the preoperative nurse teach the client about the postoperative phase? Select all that apply.
   a. The postoperative diet
   b. Deep breathing and coughing exercises
   c. Postoperative exercise of the lower extremities.
   d. The removal of dentures.
   e. Pain control techniques.
   f. The skin preparation.

Answer: b. c. e. The preoperative nurse can teach the client about deep breathing and coughing exercises, postoperative exercise of the lower extremities, and pain control techniques. The postoperative diet does not need to be discussed and the removal of dentures and skin preparation do not apply to the postoperative period.

9. What is included in the preoperative checklist?
   a. Dietary restrictions.
   b. Verification of signed surgical permit
   c. Preoperative pain medication
   d. The teaching of splinting the incision

Answer: b. As part of the preoperative checklist includes verification of signed surgical permit. Dietary restrictions, preoperative pain medication and the teaching of splinting the incision are not part of the preoperative checklist.

10. Complications of the intraoperative period include what?
    a. Hypoxia
    b. Elevated body temperature
    c. DVT
    d. Hypercoagulability state

Answer: a. Hypoxia or other respiratory problem is a complication of the intraoperative period. Hypothermia can be a complication. DVT and hypercoagulability are not complications of the intraoperative period.

11. The client is to have regional anesthesia. What do you tell the client about this type of anesthesia?
    a. The client will be intubated.
    b. A local anesthetic will be injected along the pathway of a nerve.
    c. The client will have no memory of the surgery.
    d. The surgery will take longer than with general anesthesia.

Answer: b. In regional anesthesia, a local anesthetic will be injected along the pathway of a nerve. There will be no intubation but there may be sedation. The client may have some memory of the surgery, which will take no longer than a surgery with general anesthesia.

12. The client is undergoing conscious sedation. How do you explain this to the client?
    a. There will be a better ability to tolerate unpleasant procedures while conscious.
    b. Intubation is performed after the sedation is given.
    c. No local or regional anesthesia is necessary.
    d. The client does not need an anesthetist present for the procedure.

Answer: a. The client will be better able to tolerate unpleasant procedures while conscious. There is no intubation and a local anesthetic or regional anesthetic will be used. An anesthetist will monitor the procedure.

13. The client is having local anesthetic for their surgery. How do you explain this to the client?
    a. The area along a nerve route will be anesthetized.
    b. The client will have a shorter procedure with local anesthesia.
    c. The client will have no memory of the procedure.
    d. The anesthesia will involve the area around the surgical site.

Answer: d. In local anesthesia, the area around the surgical site will be anesthetized. If the anesthetized area is along a nerve route, it is called regional anesthesia. It does not affect the length of the procedure. The client will likely remember the procedure.

Perioperative Nursing

14. The nurse tells the client about the main complications of anesthesia. What does she say? Select all that apply.
    a. Bronchospasm
    b. Hypertension
    c. Dysrhythmias
    d. Fever
    e. DVT
    f. Prolonged pain

Answer: a. b. c. Bronchospasm, hypertension, hypothermia, and dysrhythmias are all complications of anesthesia. Fever, DVT, and prolonged pain are not anesthetic complications.

15. What is the best way to reduce infection during surgery?
    a. Use povidone iodine topical solution to the affected area
    b. Give antibiotics after surgery
    c. Keep the wound free of dressings
    d. Provide adequate oxygenation

Answer: a. The use of povidone iodine or similar product will help prevent infection during surgery. Antibiotics are used at the time of surgery and not after surgery. A sterile dressing should be applied. Oxygenation is important but unrelated to risk of infection.

16. The client is undergoing conscious sedation. What things should be monitored? Check all that apply.
    a. The peripheral circulation
    b. Vital signs
    c. O2 saturation
    d. EEG
    e. The placement of the ET tube
    f. Level of consciousness

Answer: b. c. f. In conscious sedation, the vital signs, O2 saturation, and level of consciousness are monitored. The peripheral circulation is not routinely monitored nor is the placement of an ET tube or EEG.

17. You are the operating scrub nurse. What is a major part of your job?
    a. Assess level of consciousness
    b. Assess vital signs
    c. Perform instrument, sponge, and needle count
    d. Assess body temperature of client

Answer: c. As the operating scrub nurse, you are scrubbed in and cannot assess things like level of consciousness, vital signs and body temperature. You must, however, perform instrument, sponge and needle counts.

18. You are the circulating nurse in a surgery. What are some tasks you might do? Select all that apply?
    a. Manage the airway
    b. Do a sponge count
    c. Open sterile supplies
    d. Contact the post-anesthesia recovery room
    e. Assist in retraction
    f. Provide assistance for the scrub nurse

Answer: c. d. f. As the circulating nurse, you are not scrubbed in so you can't perform a sponge count or assist in retraction. You are there to assist the scrub nurse, open sterile supplies and contact the PAR when the surgery is over. The anesthetist monitors the airway.

19. You are the postoperative nurse assigned to patient care after surgery. What is your priority nursing intervention?
    a. Contacting the relatives about the surgery.
    b. Maintain a patent airway.
    c. Check the surgical dressing.
    d. Assess peripheral pulses.

Answer: b. A priority nursing intervention after surgery is to maintain a patent airway. The other choices are secondary nursing interventions and are not the priority.

20. The client is suffering from postoperative laryngospasm. What is a priority nursing intervention?
    a. Turn the client on his side.
    b. Check the vital signs
    c. Intubate the client
    d. Suction the airway of irritating secretions

Answer: d. A priority nursing intervention for laryngospasm is to suction the airway to remove irritating secretions. Vital signs and turning the client on his side is secondary. Intubation should be reserved if other methods of maintaining oxygenation fail.

21. A medication given to treat postoperative laryngospasm includes what?
    a. Inhaled racemic epinephrine
    b. Albuterol
    c. Fentanyl
    d. Corticosteroids

Answer: a. Inhaled racemic epinephrine is given to help control postoperative laryngospasm. Albuterol is given for bronchospasm. Fentanyl and corticosteroids are not indicated.

22. As a postoperative nurse, you note that the blood pressure is 20 percent less than the baseline preoperative blood pressure. What is suspected?
   a. Effects of pain on the postoperative client
   b. The giving of Fentanyl during surgery
   c. Hypovolemia from surgical blood loss
   d. Hypothermia during surgery

Answer: c. If the postoperative blood pressure is 20 percent less than the baseline preoperative blood pressure, suspect hypovolemia first.

23. You note a significant decrease in the client's postoperative blood pressure. What is a good first nursing intervention?
   a. Check the incision site
   b. Give extra fluids for resuscitation
   c. Turn the client on his left side
   d. Place the client in a semi-Fowler's position

Answer: b. If the client's blood pressure is decreased from the preoperative level, the first nursing intervention would be to increase the fluids given to the client. Placing the client in a semi-Fowler's position will make the situation worse and the other choices will not help.

24. A common cause of postoperative hypertension in a client is what?
    a. Pain
    b. Increased O2 sat
    c. Dysrhythmias
    d. Anesthesia complication

Answer: a. Pain is the most common cause of postoperative hypertension. The other choices will not result in high blood pressure.

25. The client has sinus tachycardia after surgery. What do you suspect is wrong?
    a. The patient has had an MI.
    b. The patient is suffering from a normal complication of anesthesia.
    c. The client is in pain.
    d. The client is being given too much O2.

Answer: c. Pain, anxiety, hypovolemia, and hypoxia are all possible causes of postoperative sinus tachycardia. The other choices do not cause sinus tachycardia.

26. The client has sinus tachycardia after surgery. What do you do as the postoperative nurse?
    a. Reduce the IV rate.
    b. Treat the underlying cause.
    c. Give epinephrine.
    d. Place the client in a Trendelenburg position.

Answer: b. The major intervention for postoperative sinus tachycardia is to treat the underlying cause, such as pain, hypovolemia, hypoxia, or anxiety. The other choices will not help and epinephrine will worsen the condition.

27. The client is suffering from sinus bradycardia after surgery. What is the most likely cause?
    a. Effects of general anesthesia.
    b. High spinal anesthesia
    c. Hyperthermia
    d. Acute MI

Answer: b. The most common cause of sinus bradycardia is high spinal anesthesia. Hypothermia can be a cause as well. Rarely, it is an effect of general anesthesia.

28. The client is suffering from sinus bradycardia after surgery. What is the medication of choice?
   a. Bretylium
   b. Epinephrine
   c. Atropine
   d. Norepinephrine

Answer: c. The medication of choice in sinus bradycardia is atropine. Epinephrine and norepinephrine will make the heart beat faster but are not the medication of choice. Bretylium is for arrhythmias.

29. The client is suffering from hypothermia after surgery. What is a nursing intervention?
   a. Check the vital signs
   b. Apply warm blankets
   c. Increase the IV fluids
   d. Increase client activity

Answer: b. Hypothermia is a common postoperative complication. The best treatment is to remove wet clothing and apply warm blankets.

30. The client is suffering from postoperative agitation. What is the first thing the nurse must rule out?
    a. Hypoxia
    b. Hypothermia
    c. Arrhythmia
    d. Anxiety

Answer: a. If a client is suffering from postoperative agitation, hypoxia must be ruled out before considering effects of anesthesia or anxiety.

31. The client is suffering from postoperative nausea. What should the nurse give the client?
    a. Increased fluids
    b. Zofran
    c. Atropine
    d. Increased O2

Answer: b. If the client is suffering from postoperative nausea, Zofran, Compazine, or Phenergan can be given to control the symptoms. The other choices will not help.

32. The client is at risk for gastric aspiration after surgery. What is the main risk factor for this condition?
    a. Conscious sedation
    b. Surgical pain
    c. Hypothermia
    d. Tracheal intubation

Answer: d. One of the main risk factors for aspiration is tracheal intubation. Others are obesity, pregnancy, and depressed level of consciousness.

33. A common pain control method used in the post anesthesia recovery center is the following:
    a. Massage
    b. Meditation
    c. Patient-controlled anesthesia
    d. Succinylcholine

Answer: c. Patient-controlled anesthesia is a common pain control meditation used in post anesthesia recovery.

34. The postoperative client is suffering from hypovolemia. What signs or symptoms might be present? Select all that apply.
   a. Bradycardia
   b. Tachycardia
   c. Hypertension
   d. Hypotension
   e. Cardiac arrhythmia
   f. Cool skin temperature

Answer: b. d. f. If the postoperative client is suffering from hypovolemia, the symptoms and signs most likely to be present include tachycardia, hypotension, and a cool skin temperature.

35. The postoperative client has suffered from an evisceration. What is the first nursing intervention you should consider?
   a. Replace abdominal contents
   b. Apply a sterile moist dressing to cover the affected area
   c. Increase IV fluids
   d. Turn the client to the left side

Answer: b. The first nursing intervention should be to apply a sterile moist dressing over the area and then to contact the surgeon.

36. Which postoperative finding is least worrisome?
    a. Urinary output of 30 cc/hr
    b. Respiratory rate of 20
    c. Blood pressure of 80/40
    d. Pulse of 120

Answer: a. A urinary output of 30 cc/hr is considered the minimally acceptable urine output for a postoperative patient. The other vital signs are out of acceptable range and should be reported to the physician.

37. The postoperative client has absent bowel sounds. What should the postoperative nurse do?
    a. Feed a solid meal slowly
    b. Feed liquids only
    c. Ask for permission to put an NG tube down
    d. Give a retention enema

Answer: c. A Postoperative patient with ileus may need an NG tube until bowel sounds return. You need to ask for an order from the doctor. Feeding the patient is inappropriate and a retention enema will not help.

Perioperative Nursing

38. The postoperative COPD client has an O2 Sat of 87 percent. What do you do?
    a. Talk to the anesthetist about reintubating the client.
    b. Give 100 percent O2 by rebreather mask
    c. Give albuterol
    d. Give 2-4 liters of oxygen by nasal cannula

Answer: d. The client with COPD cannot have too much oxygen or they will lose their respiratory drive to breathe. Giving 2-4 liters by nasal cannula is sufficient. Albuterol may not be necessary and reintubation is not necessary unless the client is in respiratory failure.

39. The client after surgery is at risk of deep vein thrombosis. What can you do?
    a. Ambulate the client in the post-anesthesia unit
    b. Give IV heparin
    c. Apply compression stockings
    d. Ask about inserting an intravenacaval filter

Answer: c. A person at risk for deep vein thrombosis can be taught calf pumping techniques and can have compression stockings placed. IV heparin is not necessary and may make postoperative bleeding worse. An intravenacaval filter is probably overkill unless a documented DVT exists.

40. The nurse recognizes that which of the following drugs might place the surgical client at risk for perioperative complications?
   a. Acetaminophen
   b. Aspirin
   c. Omeprazole
   d. Diphenhydramine
   e. Ibuprofen
   f. Zoloft

Answer: b. d. e. f. Aspirin can interfere with coagulation, diphenhydramine can cause symptoms suggestive of dementia, ibuprofen can interfere with coagulation and antidepressants can lower blood pressure after anesthesia.

41. Which of the following items should be included when teaching a client about an upcoming outpatient procedure?
   a. Postoperative nursing interventions
   b. Risk for postoperative complications
   c. Risks and benefits of the proposed procedure
   d. Risks and benefits of anesthetic choices

Answer: a. The nurse should discuss postoperative nursing interventions. Surgical complications, risks and benefits of the procedure, and risks/benefits of anesthetic choices are the role of the surgeon and anesthesiologist.

Perioperative Nursing

42. You are reviewing the chart of a client about to undergo general anesthesia. Which of the following is the greatest risk factor?
    a. The client who expresses anxiety about the procedure.
    b. The client who ate a snack within the last three hours
    c. The client who last smoked 24 hours ago
    d. The client who has hypertension controlled by diet and exercise

Answer: b. The client who ate just prior to surgery is at risk of aspiration. The other scenarios are of much less concern.

43. What is a priority nursing assessment when caring for a preoperative client?
    a. Ask about allergies.
    b. Verify client identity.
    c. Determine the client's nutritional status.
    d. Determine the client's neurological status.

Answer: b. The most important aspect of a preoperative nursing assessment is to verify the client's identity. The other things are of lesser importance.

44. The nurse is obtaining a history from a client at risk for malignant hyperthermia. Which of the following should the nurse assess first to get the most accurate risk assessment?
    a. Previous history of surgical complications.
    b. Drug allergies.
    c. OTC drug use.
    d. History of unexplained fevers.

Answer: a. A past history of surgical complications will alert the nurse to possible malignant hyperthermia. Drug allergies, OTC drug use, and a history of unexplained fevers do not relate to getting malignant hyperthermia.

45. The nurse is worried about a client's risk for impaired gas exchange because of ineffective airway clearance. What is a priority assessment?
    a. Respirations per minute
    b. Liters of oxygen used
    c. Decreased air movement
    d. Capillary refill

Answer: c. When it comes to ineffective air exchange, the movement of air is the most important assessment. The others are secondary.

46. The nurse cares for a postoperative client after general anesthesia. Which is a priority observation that should be reported immediately?
    a. Complaints of nausea
    b. Mild hypertension
    c. Decreased urinary output.
    d. Increasing body temperature.

Answer: d. Increasing body temperature could indicate the onset of malignant hypertension, a complication of general anesthesia. The other things are important but do not need to be reported as much as the temperature.

47. You are caring for a client who is perioperative. What is a priority nursing intervention to prevent infection during surgery?
    a. Preparation of the skin site.
    b. Maintaining hemodynamic status.
    c. Maintaining client temperature
    d. Determining estimated blood loss

Answer: a. Prepping the skin site is the most important thing to do to prevent perioperative infection. The others make no difference.

48. The nurse is caring for a client receiving conscious sedation. What is the priority item to be regularly monitored?
    a. Temperature
    b. Level of consciousness
    c. Dermatome level
    d. Urine output

Answer: b. During conscious sedation, the nurse should monitor the client's level of consciousness throughout the procedure.

49. What should the perioperative nurse monitor in evaluating ineffective thermoregulation?
    a. Cardiac rhythm
    b. Blood pressure
    c. O2 saturation
    d. Temperature

Answer: d. The client's temperature is the best way of measuring the client's thermoregulation. The other parameters do not help tell the client's thermoregulation.

50. Which is a priority nursing intervention in a postoperative client?
   a. Establishing a patent airway
   b. Maintaining adequate blood pressure
   c. Following level of consciousness
   d. Assessing pain level

Answer: a. The client must have a patent airway at all times. The other measurements take a lesser priority.

51. The client is postoperative. Which would indicate that the client has a compromised airway?
   a. A complaint of anxiety
   b. A complaint of pain
   c. A pulse oximetry reading of 90 percent
   d. Cool and clammy skin

Answer: a. The complaint of anxiety is one of the first to indicate hypoxemia. Pain is unrelated to airway problems and an O2 reading of 90 percent is acceptable. Cool and clammy skin is a nonspecific finding.

52. The postoperative client has a compromised airway. What is a priority nursing intervention for this?
    a. Reposition the client to be supine.
    b. Open the airway with a chin lift or jaw thrust.
    c. Prepare to intubate the client.
    d. Notify the surgeon.

Answer: b. The priority intervention is to try and reestablish the airway with a chin lift or jaw thrust. Intubation is likely not required.

53. What nursing measures are important in the prevention of laryngospasm?
    a. Administer atropine
    b. Reposition the client to be supine
    c. Administer high flow oxygen via mask
    d. Administer succinylcholine

Answer: d. Succinylcholine is a muscle relaxant that can reduce laryngospasm. The client can be repositioned to be in the semi-Fowler's position. Atropine will not help and high flow oxygen does not address the laryngospasm.

54. The client is immediately postoperative. What would alert the nurse that the client is becoming hypovolemic?
   a. Diastolic blood pressure of 100 mm Hg.
   b. A complaint of severe pain.
   c. A complaint of anxiety.
   d. A blood loss of 500 cc.

Answer: d. A blood loss of 500 cc would alert you to the possibility of hypovolemia. Pain, anxiety and a diastolic BP of 100 mm Hg lean toward hypertension, not a sign of hypovolemia.

55. The postoperative client develops sinus tachycardia. What is a good nursing intervention?
   a. Give warm blankets.
   b. Give atropine.
   c. Position the client in a lateral position.
   d. Manage the client's anxiety.

Answer: d. Sinus tachycardia is a manifestation of anxiety, which can be controlled. Atropine would make the situation worse and warm blankets and repositioning will not help.

56. The client has become hypothermic after surgery. The first nursing action would be what?
   a. Position the client in a lateral position.
   b. Give an analgesic.
   c. Remove wet clothing.
   d. Monitor intake and output.

Answer: c. If the client is hypothermic, wet and bloody clothing should be removed first. The other choices would not help reduce hypothermia.

57. The client is confused just after coming out of anesthesia. What is essential in determining the cause of the confusion?
   a. Check the airway.
   b. Check the cardiac rhythm
   c. Check the level of consciousness
   d. Assess the level of anxiety

Answer: a. The nurse must first assess for hypoxia by assessing the airway. The other choices are less of a priority in assessing for confusion.

Perioperative Nursing

58. The nurse is seeing a client prior to surgery. What is a specific risk factor for aspiration?
    a. Obesity
    b. Cigarette smoking
    c. An elevated sodium level
    d. A history of sleep apnea

Answer: a. An obese person has an increased pressure in the abdomen and is at an increased risk for aspiration. The other choices do not increase the risk of aspiration.

59. Which of the following is a priority for a client who has abdominal surgery and complains of pain after surgery?
    a. Monitor the blood pressure
    b. Teach the client how to splint the abdomen
    c. Reposition the client to be more comfortable
    d. Ask the client to describe the pain

Answer: d. Before treating the pain, the nurse should ask the client about the character of the pain. The rest of the choices come secondary to identifying what the pain is like.

60. A teenage client has a history of anorexia nervosa. The nurse preparing the client for abdominal surgery is most concerned about the clients risk for what?
    a. Aspiration
    b. Infection
    c. Hypovolemia
    d. Tissue perfusion

Answer: b. The client with anorexia nervosa suffers from malnutrition and problems with immunity so they are at a higher risk of infection. They are not at a higher risk of aspiration, hypovolemia or problems with tissue perfusion.

61. A client is scheduled for a surgery related to cancer exploration. The client has tears in his eyes. What would be a good nursing intervention?
    a. Contact the surgeon to alleviate the client's concerns
    b. Ask the client to describe his feelings
    c. Medicate with an analgesic
    d. Tell the client there is nothing to worry about.

Answer: b. The nurse should assess what the feelings are all about so as to provide the best intervention for the client. False reassurance will not help.

62. The client is having emergency surgery for bowel obstruction. What is the client most at risk for in the perioperative period?
    a. Infection
    b. Electrolyte imbalance
    c. Aspiration
    d. Airway obstruction

Answer: c. The client has a backing up of the intestinal contents and so is at a greater risk of aspiration. The client is not at a greater risk of infection, electrolyte imbalance or airway obstruction.

63. The client in the post anesthesia care unit after abdominal surgery complains of feeling a pop and a gush of warm fluid coming from the incision site. The nurse concludes it is from a wound dehiscence. Priority nursing interventions include what? Select all that apply.
    a. Place the client in the supine position.
    b. Get a set of vital signs
    c. Cover the wound with a sterile dressing
    d. Apply O2 at 8 l/min
    e. Contact the surgeon
    f. Increase the IV fluids

Answer: a. c. e. The client should be positioned in a supine position to avoid evisceration. A sterile dressing should be applied. The surgeon should be contacted. Vital signs are not a priority and O2/IV fluids are only to be given if necessary.

Perioperative Nursing

64. A client has a patient-controlled analgesia machine ordered. The best time to start the PCA pump is when?
    a. When the client complains of pain
    b. When the client arrives after surgery
    c. Just prior to transfer to the floor
    d. When the client shows evidence of nonverbal signs of pain

Answer: b. The PCA pump should be started as soon as the patient arrives after surgery. It shouldn't wait until the pain is already obvious.

65. Which of the following tasks can be assigned to the licensed practical nurse?
    a. Informing the client scheduled for surgery about the procedure.
    b. Instruct the client scheduled for surgery on the preop preparation.
    c. Get an informed consent from the client.
    d. Administer a preoperative intramuscular medication.

Answer: d. The LPN may give an intramuscular injection but cannot do any teaching, instructing or getting of an informed consent.

66. The postoperative client is ready to be discharged to the floor. What is a sign that the client has an adequate cardiac output?
   a. Cold, clammy skin
   b. Pale mucus membranes
   c. Normal blood pressure
   d. Pulse of 40

Answer: c. The client shows evidence of normal cardiac output with a normal pulse and blood pressure, warm skin, and pink mucus membranes.

67. The postoperative client has tenderness in the calf and swelling of the calf. What is the most appropriate nursing intervention?
   a. Apply compression stockings.
   b. Give subcutaneous heparin.
   c. Inform the surgeon.
   d. Watch for further findings.

Answer: c. The client probably already has a deep vein thrombosis and subcutaneous heparin/compression stockings are too late. It is inappropriate to wait for further findings. The surgeon should be notified.

68. The postoperative client is complaining of nausea. What does the nurse do?
    a. Notify the surgeon
    b. Give Zofran as ordered.
    c. Increase O2 to 8 liters per minute
    d. Turn the client to the side.

Answer: b. The client suffering from nausea can be given Zofran. The surgeon does not need to be notified and O2 will not help. Turning the client on the left side is acceptable if there is imminent vomiting.

69. The postoperative client is complaining of incisional pain. What is the first nursing intervention?
    a. Assess the level of pain on the pain scale.
    b. Give IV morphine.
    c. Contact the surgeon.
    d. Change the incisional dressing.

Answer: a. When the client complains of pain, the first intervention is to ask what the level of pain is on the pain scale before giving them the pain medication. The surgeon does not have to be contacted and changing the dressing will not address the pain.

70. What is the most important thing to have in place before entering surgery?
    a. Signed permit for surgery
    b. Client's dietary preferences
    c. History of past surgeries
    d. IV

Answer: a. The signed permit for surgery is the most important thing to have in place before a client enters surgery. An IV can be placed by the anesthesiologist in the surgical suite and the client's dietary preferences and list of past surgeries is less important.

71. What does the client say to indicate that he is ready for discharge from the postoperative recovery area after having general anesthesia to home?
    a. "I will drive very carefully toward home".
    b. "I can return to work later this day."
    c. "I do not need to follow up with my surgeon."
    d. "I have the surgeon's number in case I have complications."

Answer: d. The client needs to know who to call if problems arise after surgery. They cannot drive themselves home or work after general anesthesia. Follow up with the surgeon is almost always a part of the discharge plan.

Perioperative Nursing

72. What is appropriate to teach the client about pain relief after discharge from surgery?
    a. Continue the opioid pain reliever until the bottle is gone.
    b. Use non-pharmacological measures of pain control as the incision heals.
    c. Take NSAIDs for pain as soon as the client gets home.
    d. Take more opioid medication if the pain suddenly worsens.

Answer: b. The client can use non-pharmacological measures for pain control as the incision heals. Opioids should be given only when pain occurs and the bottle does not have to be finished. NSAIDs may or may not be part of pain control measures after surgery. If the pain suddenly worsens, the surgeon or postoperative unit should be notified.

73. What is a priority for the postoperative patient do in order to prevent pneumonia?
    a. Drink fluids only to prevent aspiration.
    b. Ambulate shortly after surgery.
    c. Use an incentive spirometer after surgery.
    d. Lie in a semi-Fowler's position.

Answer: c. An incentive spirometer is a priority treatment for the prevention of pneumonia. Ambulation may help but may not be possible right after surgery. Fluids can be aspirated as well as solids and the sitting position is less important than using incentive spirometry.

74. Each of the following tasks can be given to an LPN as part of intraoperative care. Select all that apply.
    a. Teaching incentive spirometry to the client.
    b. Monitor vital signs
    c. Obtain informed consent.
    d. Teach wound care to the client.
    e. Monitor intake and output.
    f. Assist with turning, coughing, and deep breathing.

Answer: b. e. f. The LPN can monitor vital signs, assist in hygiene, monitor intake and output, and assist with turning, coughing, and deep breathing. The LPN cannot obtain informed consent and cannot do activities requiring teaching to the client.

75. The patient is being discharged to home. What indicates the client has understood the oral and written instructions?
    a. "I will take more antibiotics if the wound is reddened or is draining."
    b. "I will take my temperature if I feel warm."
    c. I will inspect the wound twice daily."
    d. "I will not lift anything heavy for 48 hours after going home."

Answer: c. The client is to inspect the wound twice daily and call if the wound is reddening or draining. The temperature should be taken regularly, even if a fever is not suspected. Lifting restrictions are usually much longer than 48 hours.

76. The client needs nutritional advice before leaving the hospital after surgery. What advice do you give?
    a. Limit protein to less than 1 g/kg/day of body weight.
    b. A calorie restricted diet can be resumed if it was ongoing before surgery.
    c. Increase zinc to 4-6 mg/day
    d. Drink up to 1000 cc of fluids per day.

Answer: c. The client should be on a high protein, high calorie diet after surgery. They should take zinc, which increases wound healing. They should also drink in excess of 2000 cc of fluids per day.

77. The alcoholic client is being discharged from same day surgery. What do you advise the client to do around drinking behaviors?
    a. Taking medications with alcohol is acceptable.
    b. Go back to drinking what they had been drinking prior to surgery.
    c. Do not drink after surgery.
    d. Report signs of alcohol withdrawal syndrome to the physician promptly.

Answer: d. In some cases, the client will need to resume some alcohol to avoid withdrawal and in others, stopping drinking will promote healing. Medications should not be taken with alcohol, especially opioid infections. The client should report signs of alcohol withdrawal syndrome to the physician promptly.

78. You are discharging an elderly client after surgery. What should you warn the client most about?
    a. There will be an increase in wound infections.
    b. There will be decreased ability of the kidneys to get rid of opioids.
    c. There will be a decreased risk of fever.
    d. There will be an increased perception of pain.

Answer: b. The elderly client needs to know that there is a decreased ability of the kidneys to get rid of opioids. Pain perception may be decreased. The elderly have the same risk of wound infections and risk of fever.

79. The client is Muslim and faces surgery to remove body parts. What do you do to discuss this with the client?
    a. Tell the client it is hospital policy to discard body parts that are removed from the body.
    b. Reassure the client that diseased body parts will be left in the body.
    c. Listen to the client's concern about removal of body parts.
    d. Get a written consent for surgery that includes removal of body parts that are diseased.

Answer: c. A Muslim client will be against the removal of body parts. It is the nurse's responsibility to listen to the client's concern but to make no promises about the removal of body parts as part of the surgery. It is the surgeon's responsibility to get a written consent from the client including the disposition about the removal of body parts.

80. What is part of the informed consent for surgery?
    a. Consequences of failing to follow surgeon's orders.
    b. Risks and benefits of surgery.
    c. The name of the anesthesiologist involved in the surgery.
    d. The signature of the surgeon.

Answer: b. The informed consent should contain the name of the surgeon, the name of the proposed procedure, the risks and benefits of the surgery, consequences of not having surgery and the client's signature.

81. What is important about getting the informed consent for surgery?
    a. The informed consent can be gotten after the client has had a sedative.
    b. The informed consent can be gotten after surgery if the client has had sedation.
    c. The LPN can get the informed consent prior to surgery.
    d. The informed consent must be gotten before the client has had sedation.

Answer: d. The informed consent must be gotten by the surgeon and must be gotten before the client has received sedation. It must be gotten prior to surgery.

82. For what is informed consent not required?
    a. For the giving of oxygen during surgery.
    b. For the disposal of body parts during surgery.
    c. For the donation of organs after death.
    d. For photographing the client during surgery.

Answer: a. Informed consent is necessary for all items except the giving of oxygen during surgery.

83. A minor is having heart surgery. What is true of giving informed consent?
    a. The minor may give consent if he or she is above the age of 16.
    b. The minor may not give any informed consent.
    c. The minor may give informed consent if he or she demonstrates understanding of the consent papers.
    d. The minor may give informed consent if he or she has not been sedated.

Answer: b. Informed consent must be signed by the minor's legal guardian or parent.

84. Which of the following measures are nursing responsibilities when a client is having surgery? Select all that apply.
    a. Develop an individualized plan of care.
    b. Serve as the client's advocate.
    c. Call "time out" if a potential error is observed.
    d. Communicate the outcome of the surgery to the family.
    e. Collaborate with the healthcare team.
    f. Order the client's sedative.

Answer: a. b. c. e. The nurse's job is to develop an individualized plan of care, serve as the client's advocate, and call "time out" if a potential error is observed. The nurse must also collaborate with the healthcare team. It is the surgeon's job to communicate the outcome of the surgery to the family and to order a sedative.

85. The client is to have elective surgery. The nurse should plan with the client to schedule the surgery:
    a. If the client wishes to have the procedure done
    b. At the client's earliest convenience.
    c. Within the next two weeks.
    d. Within the next 2 days.

Answer: b. The elective surgery should be scheduled at the client's earliest convenience.

Perioperative Nursing

86. The client is to be NPO for at least 8 hours before having same day surgery. You learn that a client had a half glass of juice 3 hours prior to admission. What should you do?
    a. Report the incident to the nursing supervisor.
    b. Inform the surgery department.
    c. Notify the anesthesiologist.
    d. Reschedule the surgery.

Answer: c. Fluid restriction is designed to minimize aspiration during surgery. The anesthesiologist should be notified but it is up to the anesthesiologist to decide if the surgery should be rescheduled.

87. The client is anxious before surgery. As the preoperative nurse, you should do what?
    a. Give an anti-anxiety agent.
    b. Describe the procedure to the client.
    c. Reassure the client about the surgeon's capabilities.
    d. Encourage verbalization of feelings.

Answer: d. Surgery is an anxiety-provoking event and the client should be offered the opportunity to verbalize his or her feelings of anxiety.

88. The client is receiving atropine prior to surgery. What is the intended outcome of this medication?
    a. Constrict the pupils.
    b. Stimulate the central nervous system.
    c. Decrease cardiac output.
    d. Suppress oral secretions.

Answer: d. In the case of surgery, atropine is often given to suppress oral and respiratory secretions. It decreases the activity of the central nervous system, dilates the pupils and increases cardiac output.

89. The client is receiving Tagamet prior to surgery. What is the intended outcome of giving this drug?
    a. To decrease volume of gastric secretions.
    b. To decrease the pH of gastric secretions.
    c. To reduce the amount of anesthetic needed.
    d. To dispel unpleasant sensations around the procedure.

Answer: a. Tagamet can decrease the volume of gastric secretions. It increases the pH of gastric secretions and does nothing to affect the amount of anesthesia needed.

90. The client arrives in the operating room wearing two post earrings on each eyebrow. What should be done?
   a. Ask the client to remove the earrings and place them in a labelled container.
   b. Call a nurse on the med-surge unit to remove the earrings and give them to a family member.
   c. Remind the anesthetist to remove the earrings when the client is anesthetized.
   d. Secure the earrings with paper tape.

Answer: a. The client should remove the earrings and they should be placed in a labelled container. They should not be placed in the hands of a family member nor is it the anesthetist's responsibility to remove the jewelry. The jewelry must be removed.

91. The nurse notices that a cart brought to transport the client has a nonfunctioning clasp on the safety belt. What should be done?
   a. Call the Safety/Security Department to report the problem.
   b. Use a draw sheet to secure the client during transport.
   c. Contact the engineering department to repair the clasp.
   d. Request a new cart with a functioning clasp.

Answer: d. The nurse is responsible for the safety of the client and should request that a new cart with a functioning clasp be ordered.

92. The surgeon is checking the x-ray of a client who is in the operating room for a lung lobectomy. The nurse notices that the name on the x-ray is not that of the client's. What should the nurse do?
    a. Call the x-ray tech to take another x-ray.
    b. Call the surgeon aside to ask to have the x-ray checked.
    c. Look for the correct x-ray.
    d. Call a time out.

Answer: d. Whenever a potential error is discovered, it is up to the nurse to call a time out until the problem can be sorted out.

93. The client is receiving a large volume of packed RBCs during surgery. The nurse should observe the client for hypocalcemia because:
    a. Extra calcium is needed during stressful events.
    b. Anesthesia causes hypocalcemia.
    c. Hypo-perfusion to the parathyroid glands affects calcium levels.
    d. The preservative in packed red blood cells binds with calcium.

Answer: d. Citrate is used as a preservative in packed RBCs and can chelate with calcium in the client's system, resulting in hypocalcemia.

94. The client had a partial gastrectomy 24 hours ago and has a nasogastric tube in place. The expected outcome of using a nasogastric tube after a partial gastrectomy is what?
   a. To assess the pH of gastric secretions.
   b. To remove stomach contents.
   c. To delay peristalsis until healing takes place.
   d. To assess the characteristics of drainage at the anastomotic site.

Answer: b. The nasogastric tube is in place to remove stomach contents that might put extra pressure on the incision inside the stomach.

95. Three days after a cholecystectomy, a client states that he feels like his stomach is going to burst. He is taking a regular diet. After determining the vitals are stable, in which order does the client do the following to help the client?
   a. Position the client on the right side.
   b. Offer 120 cc of hot liquids.
   c. Auscultate the bowel sounds.
   d. Encourage ambulation.

Answer: c. b. a. d. The nurse should first listen for bowel sounds and then give hot liquids to stimulate peristalsis. Positioning the patient on the right side will allow air to rise from the transverse colon, making it easier to be expelled. Finally, ambulation can encourage peristalsis.

96. The nurse sees that the client is restless during the immediate postoperative period. What should the nurse do first?
    a. Give a sedative.
    b. Offer ice chips.
    c. Give oxygen.
    d. Apply wrist restraints.

Answer: c. Restlessness in the immediate postoperative period could mean the client is hypoxic. Oxygen should be given first before any other intervention.

97. A nurse listens to the client's breath sounds on the fourth postoperative day and hears a loud, low-pitched, rumbling sound on expiration. What should the nurse do first?
    a. Give oxygen.
    b. Encourage coughing.
    c. Request an order for incentive spirometry.
    d. Reposition the client to a high Fowler position.

Answer: b. The client should first be encouraged to turn and cough in order to loosen secretions that might be causing the sounds heard.

98. During the extended postoperative period after an abdominal hysterectomy, the nurse notes a urine output of 20 cc/hr. What should the nurse do?
   a. Consider this to be normal.
   b. Evaluate the client's fluid intake.
   c. Prepare the client to be returned to the operating room.
   d. Consult the urologist.

Answer: b. By several day's out from surgery, the intake and output should be equal. The first thing to do is to assess the client's fluid intake before consulting anyone or returning to surgery.

99. On the first day after abdominal surgery, the nurse notices an absence of bowel sounds. What should the nurse do first?
   a. Encourage the client to use the patient-controlled analgesia pump more often.
   b. Ask another nurse to validate the findings.
   c. Encourage the client to take more ice chips.
   d. Document the findings in the client's medical record.

Answer: d. Bowel sounds are usually not heard for the third or fourth postoperative day after surgery so an absence of bowel sounds is to be expected. Document these findings in the client's record.

Perioperative Nursing

100. Before nonemergency surgery, the client needs to give informed consent. Which of the following is the responsibility of the nurse?
   a. Obtain informed consent.
   b. Explain the surgical procedure.
   c. Verify that the client understands the consent form.
   d. Inform the client about surgical risks.

Answer: c. The surgeon is responsible for explaining the surgical procedure, informing the client of the surgical risks, and obtaining the informed consent. As the client's advocate, the nurse can verify that the client understands what is on the consent form.

101. The nurse is verifying that the client has given consent for surgery. For the consent to be valid, there must be adequate disclosure of which of the following? Select all that apply.
   a. Nursing care plan in the post-anesthesia care unit.
   b. Purpose of the proposed treatment.
   c. Risks and benefits of the surgical procedure.
   d. Outcome of the surgery.
   e. Side effects of anesthetics.
   f. Name of the anesthetist.

Answer: b. c. For the surgical consent to be valid, it must list the purpose of the proposed treatment and the risks and benefits of the procedure. Side effects of anesthesia, surgical outcome, the name of the anesthetist, and the nursing plan of care are not part of the surgical consent form.

Perioperative Nursing

102. The nurse receives a call that a client is being transferred from the post-anesthesia recovery unit to the floor. What should the nurse do first when the client arrives?
   a. Assess the patency of the airway.
   b. Assess the drains in the client for patency.
   c. Check the dressing for bleeding.
   d. Compare the vital signs with those in the post-anesthesia recovery unit.

Answer: a. The patency of the client's airway is most critical as without it the patient cannot survive. This should take precedence over other client measurements and observations.

103. A client has undergone lab work prior to getting surgery. Which lab value should the nurse report to the surgeon as it might result in delay of the procedure?
   a. Sodium of 141 mEq/L
   b. Hemoglobin 8 g/dL
   c. Platelets 210,000 mm^3
   d. Creatinine 0.8 mg/dL

Answer: b. A hemoglobin of 8 g/dL is much too low and might result in the postponement of the surgical procedure. The other lab values are within normal limits.

Conclusion

I hope you received a ton of value from this book. Remember, practice makes perfect so you will have to repeat these readings.

If you enjoyed this book, would you be kind enough to leave a review on Amazon? Your positive review can help others to see what kinds of helpful resources are out there!

Thank you and good luck on your medical endeavors!

- Chase Hassen

Nurse Superhero

Highly Recommended Books for Success

1. <u>NCLEX: Cardiovascular System : 105 Nursing Practice and Rationales to Easily Crush the NCLEX!</u>

2. <u>NCLEX: Emergency Nursing : 105 Practice Questions and Rationales to Easily Crush the NCLEX!</u>

3. <u>Lab Values: 137 Values You Know to Easily Pass The NCLEX!</u>

4. <u>EKG Interpretation: 24 Hours or Less to Easily Pass the ECG Portion of the NCLEX!</u>

5. <u>Fluid and Electrolytes: 24 Hours or Less to Absolutely Crush the NCLEX Exam!</u>

6. <u>Nursing Careers: Easily Choose What Nursing Career Will Make Your 12 Hour Shift a Blast!</u>

7. <u>Night Shift: 10 Survival Tips for Nurses to Get Through The Night!</u>

8. NCLEX: Endocrine System : 105 Nursing Practice Questions and Rationales to EASILY Crush the NCLEX!

And **MUCH MUCH MORE**! Visit my amazon author page to see more at http://amzn.to/1HCtfSy

Made in the USA
San Bernardino, CA
12 November 2017